KAHINUI

An
Ancient Hawaiian
Healing and
Relaxation
Technique

Roger C. Kliesh ND PHD

ISBN: 9781675109236

DEDICATION

In memory of my sweet Malana
with deepest thanks for her love
and patience.

KAHINUI
Loosely translated as
"Good for Everyone."

ACKNOWLEDGMENTS

My sincere thanks to those that have shared their time and knowledge with me.

INTRODUCTION

When you bump your elbow, what is your response? You grab it and hold it. When a baby is upset what does a mother do? She holds and caresses it. When an animal hurts itself, it rests and licks its wounds. When a priest gives a person a blessing, they gently touch them during the blessing. Touching to relieve stress or pain, to balance the body energy, is a natural response in all animals; including the human animal. The basic principle at work here is that energy flows where attention goes.

What I offer you in this little book is an ancient energy balancing system developed in Hawai'i, similar to Reiki, but unlike that deeply structured technique it does not require any form of attunements or the knowledge of special symbols. Best of all, it is freely available to everyone.

I learned this technique during the six years I lived on The Big Island of Hawai'i and studied with several different kahuna. E 'olu'olu (please enjoy).

PROCEDURE

Please understand that the person who is receiving this procedure does not need to dis-robe for this process to be effective. I have merely shown the person in silhouette so that the positions and energy points were more easily seen and understood.

For your own benefit as well as protection, I suggest that before starting this technique you explain to the person that you are going to try to help them relax, and then also ask them for permission to touch them.

This is the general configuration of your hands while you are doing KAHINUI. Please be relaxed and breathe deeply and softly with your mental focus on your hands.

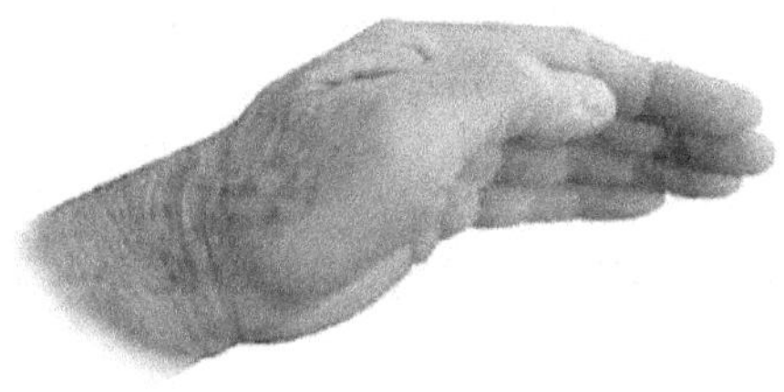

To begin the first stage of KAHINUI have the person you are helping to relax lay face down and you stand at their feet.

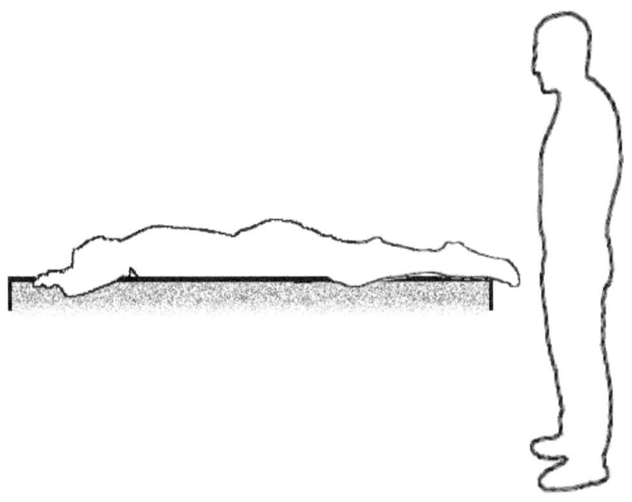

Place your relaxed hands palm down at the locations and your finger-tips closely over the points, concentrate on your hands and you will feel pulses. Focus on your hands and you will become aware that the pulses are slightly different in each hand. This is because what you are feeling is not your own blood pulse nor the blood pulse of the person you are working on. What you are feeling is an energy pulse in the body of the person. As you focus on your hands and the points you are over, the pulses will begin to synchronize with each other. This is an indication that the person's body energy is beginning to become balanced.

When the pulses feel balanced in both of your hands, move to the persons left side and continue to the next set of points. Place your right hand on 3 and your left hand on 4. When these two points are balanced maintain your energy contact with point 3 and move your left hand, balancing each point through 17, moving along the left side of the person.

After completing the entire series of energy points and you are back at numbers 2-3 you should still be on the left side of the person. Now move to stand back at the persons feet and do the 1-2 points again. When you feel that the energy is balanced at these points you can gently draw your hands away completing the full first stage of KAHINUI.

Hand positions

R	L
1	2
2	3
3	4
3	5
3	6
3	7
3	8
3	9
3	10
3	11
3	12
3	13
3	14
3	15
3	16
3	17
2	3
1	2

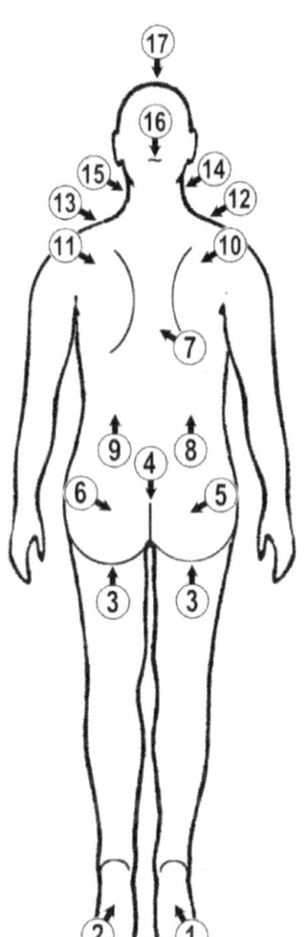

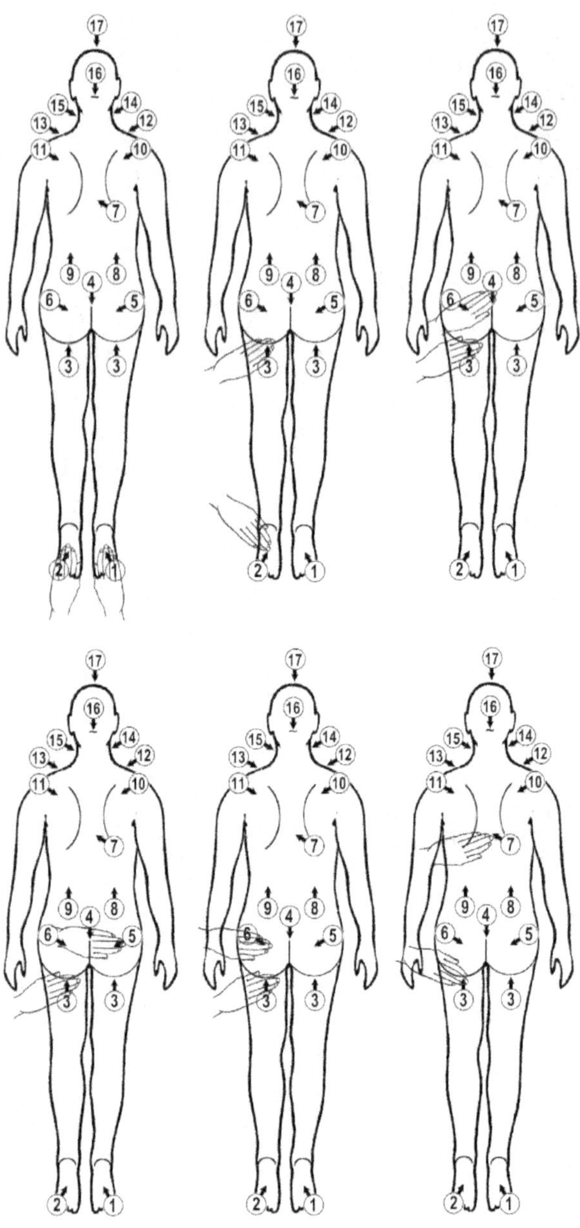

On page 6 are illustrations of the first six hand positions.

For the second stage of Kahinui, have the person you are relaxing lay face up and you stand at their feet.

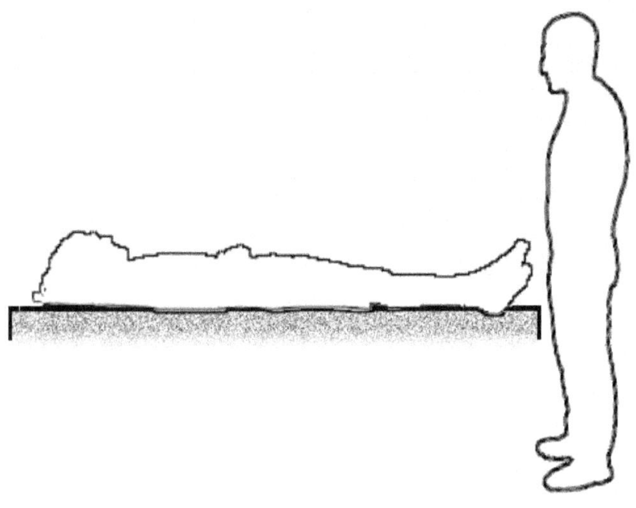

Follow the same energy pulse balancing technique as you did in stage one.

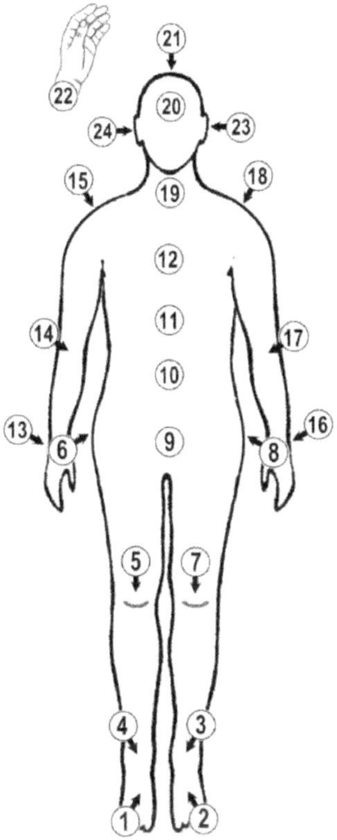

Hand positions

R	L
2	1
1	3
3	4
4	5
7	5
5	6
8	6
9	6
9	10
10	11
11	12
13	12
13	14
14	15
16	14
16	17
17	18
18	19
19	20
23	20
23	24
21	24

21 22 (this left hand is held open at your own left shoulder level)

R	L
13	21
5	13
4	5
1	4
2	1

7-3-toe   5-4-toe
(this is a knee to toe stroke)

The following is the procedure for the third stage of the KAHINUI technique.

Have the person sitting with you standing behind them.

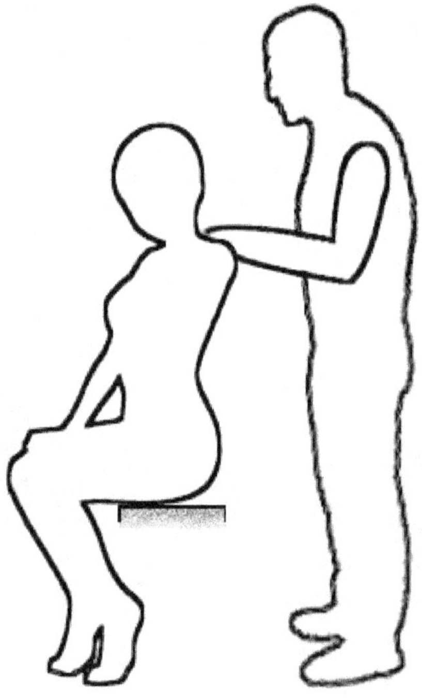

Place your open hands on the back of the shoulders with fingers up and the thumbs on the first two points (1 1) on the middle of the upper back.

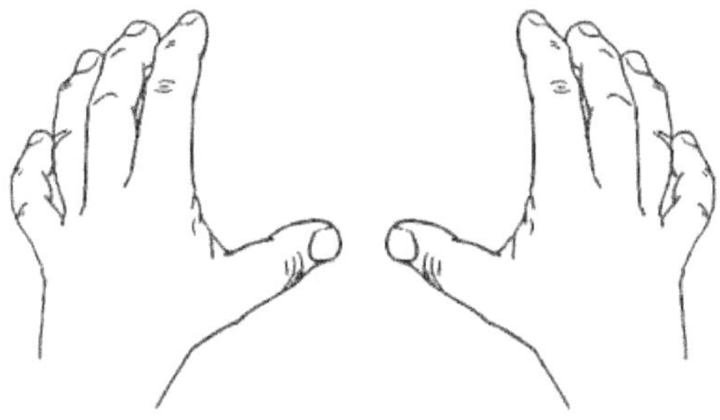

Press thumbs in firmly and hold for a count of three. Slide your open hands down to the second pair of points and press in with your thumbs. Repeat this process continuing to do the same to all the points. Repeat the entire procedure 3 times.

These are the hand locations for KAHINUI stage three energy balancing with the person sitting. This can also be done with the person standing, but it is more effective if they are in a relaxed sitting position.

L	R
1	1
2	2
3	3
4	4
5	5

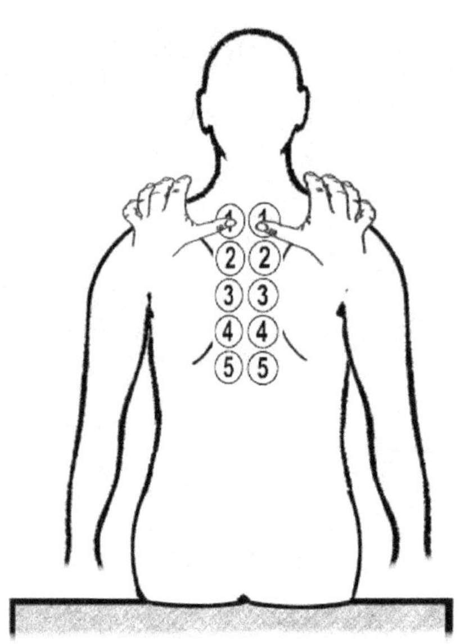

After all 5 points have been done three times, place your hands on the shoulders at the neck and then gently stroke outward and down over the arms to the elbows; do this three times. That's it. Be sure to have the person sit still for a moment or two before they stand up.

Note: This portion of KAHINUI can also be administered singularly as a quick stress reliever and relaxer.

KAHINUI

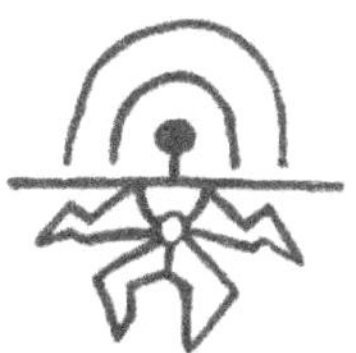

ABOUT THE AUTHOR

Roger C. Kliesh: Roger is trained in a broad mix of the holistic healing arts. His credentials include:
PhD in Holistic Nutrition; Doctor of Naturopathy; Homeopathic Practitioner; Master Herbalist; Reiki Master; and Certified Feng Shui Practitioner.

For many years Roger successfully operated a Holistic Healing Center in Florida where he positively impacted the lives of hundreds of people by helping them improve their health. Also, through his efforts and his example, many aspiring healers were introduced to the concepts and principles of traditional Naturopathy. In meeting the needs of others Roger found his pathway to universal knowledge.

This pursuit of wisdom and his passion for subtle energy knowledge led him to move to the Big Island of Hawai'i where he was privileged to study with Hawaiian kupuna. His interests then led him to Honduras where he studied local herbology and Mayan philosophy. His adventures have now brought him full circle to Florida.

BOOKS by Roger Kliesh

The Gold of Atlantis
A tale of romance, Adventure, and Intrigue.
ISBN-13: 978-1975788612

Paule and Lani flee across the Caribbean, sometimes just one frantic step ahead of their trackers. They've discovered Atlantis and its fantastic source of energy. Every exciting moment, they avoid being ruthlessly destroyed by the demented power structures of the world that are trying to destroy them and their discovery. With the astonishing help of a super-geek friend they barely stay ahead of vengeful destruction.

Balance: the Art of Wellness
(collectors copies only)

Mysteries of the Mayan Calendar
Past, Present, and Future.
ISBN-13: 978-1979875073

The ancient Maya understood that KIN (Mayan word for a day) was the primary cycle of life and that the cosmos and this Earth within it move in cycles that are flexible and infinite in their repetition. They created their calendars to track these cycles, plan their daily activities, record their history, and consider events of the future. Even today, the elders that maintain the Maya culture are called Day Keepers.

To Catch a Lightning-bug
The Short Biography of Morada
ISBN-13: 978-1530295005

This book is about Morada and the philosophy of her life, which will soon end. As she explains how and why she is where she is, you may find the story a little graphic only because she intended it to be informative; you will also find that it is entertaining.

The Power of Expectation
How Subliminal Expectation Controls our Lives
ISBN-13: 978-1981243624

What's in a name? The letters S-E are the initials of the system discussed in this amazing book and becoming aware of it can determine our ability to create a joyful and abundant reality. The SE is the energy field that drives our creativity through our Subliminal Expectations. You've probably heard someone say "You get what you expect."

When we understand our SE, it becomes our most powerful means of positive creation. If we live our lives in ignorance of the SE, it is our major cause of distress.

The concept explained here is refined from almost 40 years of accumulated knowledge. This book offers you an easily understood and effective explanation of how we create our reality, and how to change that if we choose. This is not a religious work, not a spiritual work, nor a metaphysical work. It is a work in practicality.

Traditional Remedies of Central America
ISBN-13: 978-1981190027

Bienvenidos!
Welcome to this exciting and informative little book. I'd like to share a collection of home-style remedies with you. Some may look familiar; others will be unique and intriguing. Please enjoy!

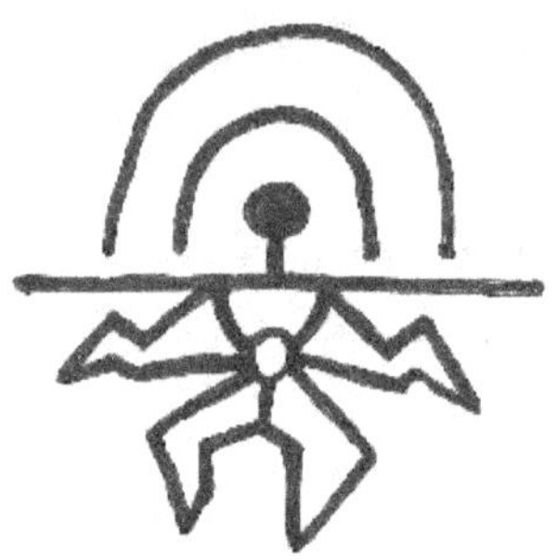